Illustrated Pocketbook
of
Prostatic Diseases

An
Illustrated Pocketbook
of
Prostatic Diseases

Roger S. Kirby, MD, FRCS(Urol), FEBU

Professsor of Urology
St. George's Hospital, London, UK

The Parthenon Publishing Group
International Publishers in Medicine, Science & Technology

A CRC PRESS COMPANY
BOCA RATON   LONDON   NEW YORK   WASHINGTON, D.C.

Published in the USA by
The Parthenon Publishing Group
345 Park Avenue South, 10th Floor
New York, NY 10010, USA

Published in the UK and Europe by
The Parthenon Publishing Group Limited
23–25 Blades Court, Deodar Road
London SW15 2NU, UK

Library of Congress Cataloging-in-Publication Data

Data available on application

British Library Cataloguing in Publication Data

Data available on application

ISBN 1-84214-056-6

Typeset by Martin Lister Publishing Services, Carnforth, UK
Printed and bound by Butler & Tanner Ltd, Frome and London

Contents

Introduction

After years of comparative obscurity, the prostate gland has finally emerged from the shadows into the full glare of media publicity. Until a few years ago, most of the public were only dimly aware of the work of urologists – many confused them with neurologists and thought they dealt with brain disorders! Suddenly, all that has changed; now barely a week goes by without some media focus on the prostate and its diseases.

What lies behind this startling change? Increasing life expectancy has swollen the ranks of men beyond middle age. These individuals have a 43% risk of symptoms of benign prostatic hyperplasia (BPH) and a 9% chance of being diagnosed as suffering from prostate cancer. Prostatitis, the third component of the triad of diseases considered in this Pocketbook, ranks among the 20 most frequent causes of outpatient visits to urologists, and is a cause of significant morbidity among sufferers.

Although not always life-threatening, prostate diseases are often associated with a significant reduction of quality of life. The ever-swelling ranks of men beyond middle-age are increasingly reluctant to accept restrictions on their activities as they grow older. For the first time, a lobby is developing to press for a more active approach to prostate disease from governments, insurers and healthcare providers. Prostate diseases are now acknowledged as an important component of men's health and worthy of proper scrutiny and active treatment.

In this volume, the anatomy and physiology of the normal prostate are described. The molecular basis of BPH, prostate cancer and prostatitis is illustrated. We conclude with the pathology, means of diagnosis and treatment of these most prevalent disorders. We hope that the result will be of value to all those caring for the very many men who suffer from prostate problems.

Anatomy

The lobar concept of the anatomy of the prostate originally suggested by Lowsley[1] is no longer helpful. The accepted view today is that of McNeal[2], who suggested that the prostate consists of three distinct zones: a central zone (CZ); transition zone (TZ); and peripheral zone (PZ; Figures 1 and 2). The TZ is the site of development of BPH, whereas the PZ is where both prostatitis and prostate cancer mainly occur[3].

The explanation for these contrasting zonal susceptibilities to different diseases probably lies in their different phylogenetic origins. In primates, the gland is divided into a cranial prostate and a caudal prostate (Figure 3). Their fusion in humans creates a single gland which completely encircles the urethra, but the different zonal pathological tendencies underline their disparate origins.

In humans, the prostate is composed of approximately 20 arborizing glandular structures which are spread out into a matrix of fibromuscular

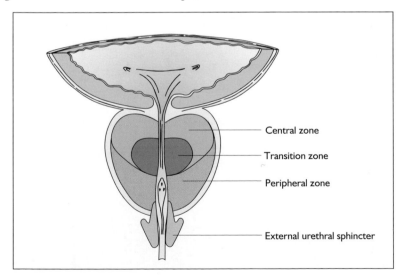

Figure 1 The prostate is composed of three distinct zones: the peripheral zone (PZ); the transition zone (TZ); and the central zone (CZ) (anterior view). Prostate cancer most commonly originates in the PZ; in contrast, BPH almost exclusively affects the TZ and periurethral tissues

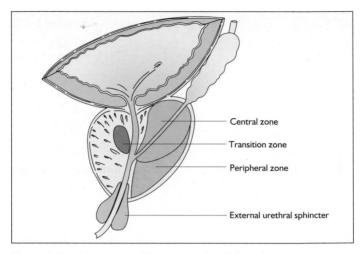

Figure 2 The three zones of the prostate (sagittal view)

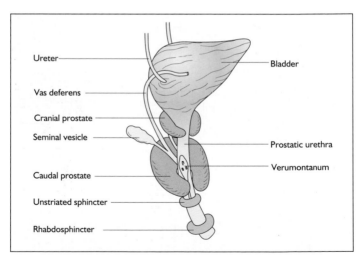

Figure 3 In primates, the prostate is divided into a caudal prostate and a cranial prostate. In phylogenetic terms, the cranial prostate is thought to be the precursor of the central zone, whereas the caudal prostate is considered the precursor of the peripheral zone. In humans, the two structures are fused, but the zones are susceptible to different disease processes

stroma (Figure 4). Current evidence suggests that newly formed epithelial cells are mainly located in the distal segments of the glands. In the mid-acinar portions, epithelial cells are tall and columnar, and perform a secretory role (Figure 5). In the distal ductal portions, the epithelial cells are lower in height and exhibit frequent apoptosis (programmed cell death).

The major function of prostatic epithelium is to elaborate prostate-specific antigen (PSA; Figure 6). Discovered by Wang et al.[4], PSA is a single-chain glycoprotein consisting of 237 amino acids. The gene encoding PSA is located on chromosome 19, close to the androgen response element (ARE). Transcription of this gene is stimulated by the formation of intracellular dihydrotestosterone (DHT). Messenger RNA (mRNA) encoding PSA is then translated into a glycoprotein protease (of the kallikrein family) which

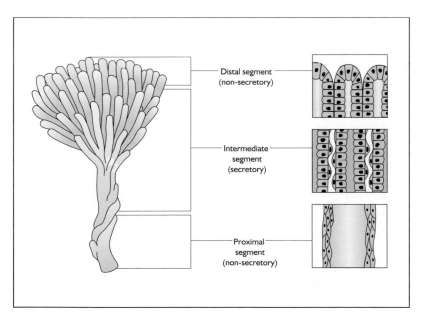

Figure 4 Prostatic ducts arborize throughout the gland and terminate in acini which secrete, among other things, prostate-specific antigen (PSA) into the lumina and thence into the prostatic urethra. New cells are formed in the distal segments of the ducts, whereas the intermediate section is secretory in function. In the proximal segment, epithelial cells become flattened and undergo programmed cell death (apoptosis)

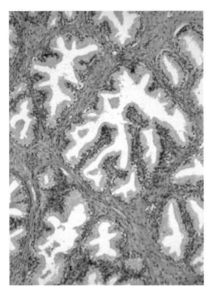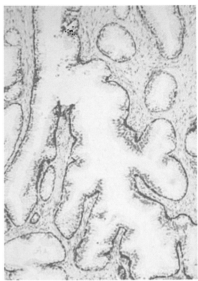

Figure 5 Normal prostatic acini are lined by tall columnar cells with a peripheral basal cell layer (left; H & E). The latter cell layer is more easily seen when stained immuno-cytochemically by antibody LP34 against cytokeratins of high molecular weight (right)

liquefies semen after ejaculation and is released into the lumina of the prostatic acini.

Normally, only a small proportion (around 0.1%) of the total PSA output is absorbed across the basal cell layer and through the basement membrane into the bloodstream; serum levels are usually below 4 ng/ml (Figure 7).

However, prostatic diseases, and especially prostate cancer, which result in damage to the integrity of the basal cell layer and basement membrane, are associated with serum PSA levels greater than this value; thus, PSA is able to serve as a marker for pathological changes[5]. In addition, increasing age in itself is associated with gradual progressive PSA elevation[6] (Figure 8), probably due to increasing leakage of PSA across the basement membrane.

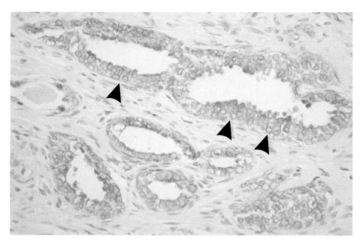

Figure 6 Prostate-specific antigen (PSA) can be demonstrated in luminal cells by immunocytochemical staining. The basal cells (arrowed) can be shown not to contain PSA

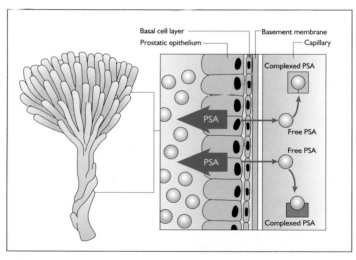

Figure 7 Prostate-specific antigen (PSA) is a glycoprotein protease secreted by the epithelium of prostatic acini. Most of the PSA produced eventually reaches the ejaculate wherein its function is to liquefy semen. Around 0.1% of the total volume, however, is absorbed across the basement membrane to reach the bloodstream, where it is mainly bound by either antichymotrypsin (ACT) or α_2-macroglobulin (α_2-MG)

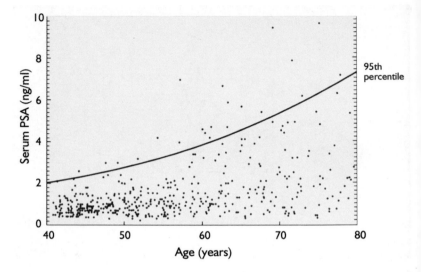

Figure 8 Probably as a result of age-associated leakiness of the basal cell layer and basement membrane, but also because of benign prostatic hyperplasia (BPH), serum PSA values tend to increase with age

Stromal-to-epithelial ratios

The ratio of stroma to epithelium in the normal and hyperplastic prostate has been studied quantitatively by both Bartsch et al.[7] and Shapiro et al.[8]. Morphometric data suggest that the normal prostate is composed of approximately 40% smooth muscle (Figure 9) and 20% glandular epithelium. In BPH, particularly of the stromal variety, the smooth muscle component may be as much as 60% of the total volume. Between individuals, however, there is wide variation with marked tissue heterogeneity even within the same gland.

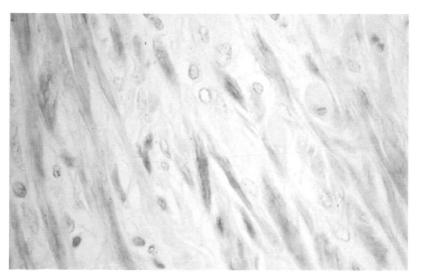

Figure 9 A considerable proportion of the prostate is composed of stroma rather than epithelium, the dominant constituent of which is smooth muscle cells, as exemplified by this section of normal prostate (immunocytochemical preparation)

Innervation of the prostate

To explain the innervation of the prostate, it is necessary to describe briefly the neurophysiology of continence and micturition. The bladder and urethra are innervated by three sets of nerves: the sympathetic, from T10 to L1 spinal levels; the parasympathetic, from sacral spinal segments S2 to S4; and the pudendal nerve, which carries somatic innervation from S2 to S4 (Figure 10).

During bladder-filling, sensory nerve endings detect progressive stretching of the bladder wall and convey information via the parasympathetic nerves to the spinal cord and brain. Increasing activity in these nerves produces a progressive reflex contraction in the bladder neck and prostatic urethra as well as in the external urethral sphincter, thereby maintaining urinary continence.

When the bladder volume reaches 300–500 ml, an awareness of the need to void develops, although true bladder contractions should not occur until a socially convenient time arrives. Voluntary voiding is accomplished as a

15

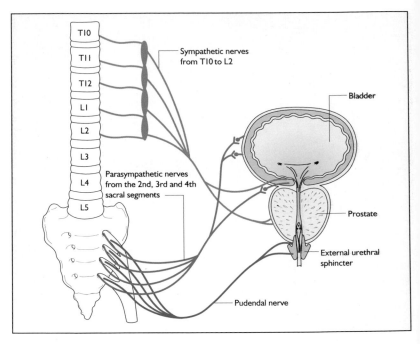

Figure 10 Three sets of nerves control continence and micturition. The parasympathetic system induces detrusor contraction during voiding whereas the sympathetic nerves and pudendals (somatic) maintain prostatic and urethral muscle tone to maintain continence

result of a barrage of impulses down the parasympathetic nerves to the detrusor muscle (Figure 11). The neurotransmitter acetylcholine (ACh) is released, which binds to muscarinic receptors on detrusor smooth muscle cells to produce coordinated contraction of the bladder body.

At the same time, neural impulses passing down the sympathetic and pudendal motor fibers cease momentarily, thereby allowing relaxation of the normally tonically contracted bladder neck, prostatic urethra and external sphincter. Bladder pressure rises, the bladder neck funnels and urine flow commences, achieving a maximum flow rate of more than 15 ml/s with a maximum detrusor pressure of less than 40 cm of water in normal men.

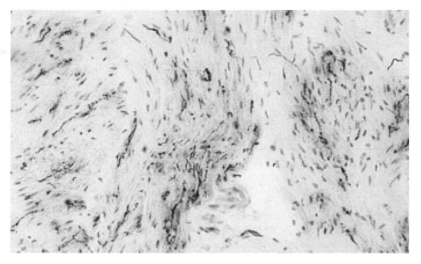

Figure 11 The parasympathetic innervation of the detrusor muscle can be demonstrated by use of a special stain for acetylcholinesterase. Nerve fibers are stained brown and can be seen in association with the detrusor smooth muscle cells

Provided that the urethra is unobstructed, bladder contraction continues until emptying is complete; urethral and bladder neck tonus is then re-established and the bladder-filling cycle begins again.

The main functional innervation of the prostate is through the sympathetic (noradrenergic) nervous system (Figure 12), although acetylcholinesterase-containing (presumably parasympathetic) and non-adrenergic, non-cholinergic (NANC) nerve fibers are also present.

Intraneural recordings from peripheral nerves elsewhere in the body reveal continuous waves of motor impulses from small unmyelinated so-called C fibers, which subserve tonic vasomotor tone. Presumably, a similar situation occurs within the prostate; it has been proposed that bladder outflow obstruction due to BPH may be related to chronic overactivity of the sympathetic nervous system in the same way that chronic overactivity of vasomotor fibers may result in systemic hypertension.

17

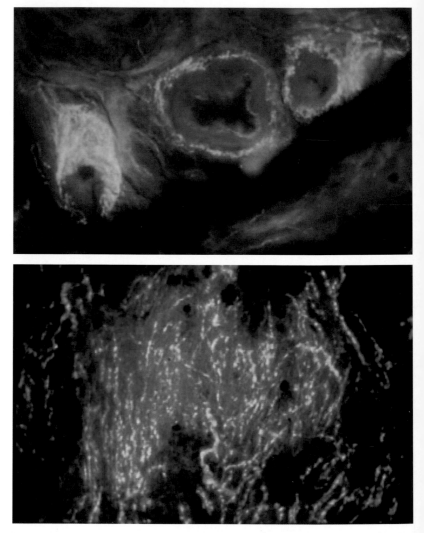

Figure 12 Immunofluorescence staining of sympathetic nerve endings in the wall of a blood vessel (upper). These nerves are responsible for the maintenance of vaso-constrictor tone. Catecholamine immunofluorescence staining demonstrates the rich sympathetic innervation of the prostate (lower). Sympathetic nerves control prostatic smooth muscle tone and can be modulated by α_1-adrenoceptor blockers

Ejaculatory function

Apart from its important role in maintaining urinary continence, prostatic and bladder neck sympathetic innervation is also essential for ejaculation. Erectile function, by contrast, is subserved by parasympathetic fibers which pass in the so-called neurovascular bundles of Walsh lying posterolateral to the prostate; these fibers are capable of producing vasodilatation within the corpora cavernosa[9] (Figure 13). In this periprostatic location, these nerves are vulnerable to injury during either radical prostatectomy or radical cystoprostatectomy for the surgical excision of urological malignancy (Figure 14). Other types of pelvic surgery may also damage erectile function.

At the time of ejaculation, a synchronized sequence of sympathetically induced contractions develops in the vasa deferentia, seminal vesicles and prostatic smooth muscle itself. This activity delivers a mixture of fluid from

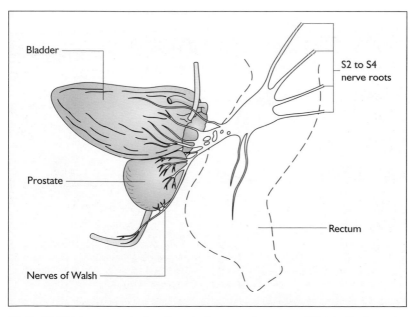

Figure 13 The neurovascular bundles, also known as the nerves of Walsh after the urologist who first described them, convey nerve impulses and blood to the corpora cavernosa and thereby subserve penile erection. Their location posterolateral to the prostate renders them vulnerable during radical prostatectomy or cystoprostatectomy

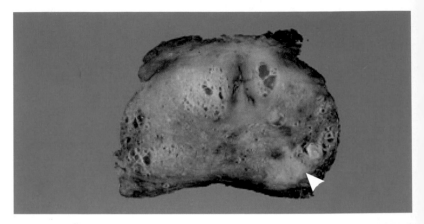

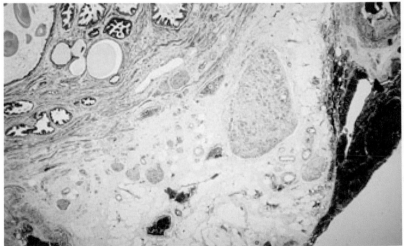

Figure 14 Transverse section from a radical prostatectomy specimen. The cancer is located posteriorly (arrowed; upper). On histology (lower), the neurovascular bundles can be seen lying posterolaterally, where they are susceptible to malignant infiltration. Prostatic intraepithelial neoplasia is present, but cancer is not seen at this level. (H & E)

the seminal vesicles, semen from the vasa and fluid containing PSA from the prostate into the prostatic urethra via openings in the verumontanum. Tight closure of the bladder neck then creates a 'pressure chamber' within the prostate such that, when reflex relaxation of the external sphincter occurs in conjunction with pulsatile contractions of the bulbocavernous muscles, antegrade ejaculation results (Figure 15).

Surgical procedures on the prostate, such as transurethral resection of the prostate (TURP), which render the bladder neck incompetent, interfere with this pressure chamber effect and often result in retrograde ejaculation.

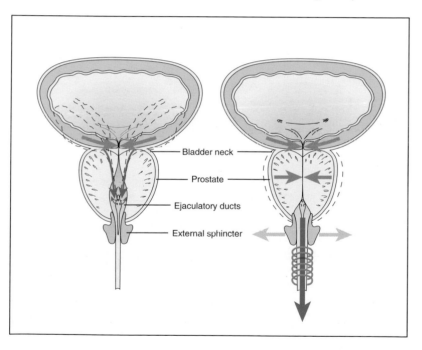

Figure 15 The mechanism of ejaculation is a complex neurophysiological process which involves contraction of the prostate and seminal vesicles, which empty their contents into the prostatic urethra. At the same time, the bladder neck closes to create a 'pressure chamber'. Rhythmic relaxation of the distal urethral sphincter and contractions of the bulbocavernous muscles around the bulbar urethra result in a pulsatile expulsion of a mixture of seminal and prostatic fluid

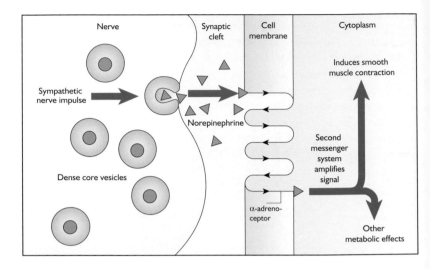

Figure 16 Norepinephrine (NE) acts as the main signal molecule at the adrenoceptor located on the cell membrane of prostatic smooth muscle cell. NE is stored in dense-core vesicles within sympathetic nerve terminals. The arrival of an impulse at the nerve ending stimulates the release of NE, which then diffuses across the synaptic gap to interact with postsynaptic adrenoceptors, mainly of the α_1 subtype

Adrenoceptor signal transduction

The neurotransmitter molecule norepinephrine (noradrenaline; NE) is located within dense-core vesicles in sympathetic nerve terminals located within the prostate. The arrival of nerve impulses at the nerve endings provokes NE release by a process of fusion of these vesicles with the cell membrane of the nerve endings. NE then diffuses across the synaptic gap to bind with either α_1-adrenoceptors, situated on the membrane of prostatic smooth muscle cells, or α_2-adrenoceptors, located on the nerve terminal itself (Figure 16). These α_2-adrenoceptors are autoregulatory in function and their blockade, by non-specific α-adrenoceptor blockers such as phenoxybenzamine, results in raised circulatory catecholamine levels with a consequent increase in side-effects such as tachycardia and palpitations.

The α_1-adrenoceptors located on the smooth muscle cell membrane are now known to consist of seven transmembrane domains and are linked intracellularly to a guanidine nucleotide binding protein (G-protein)

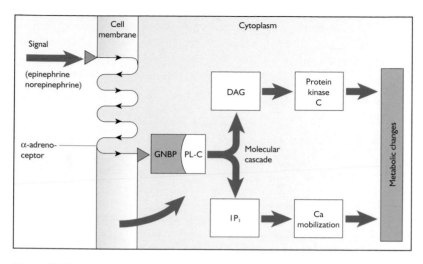

Figure 17 Signal transduction at the adrenoceptor is coupled to guanidine nucleotide binding protein (GNBP), the so-called G-protein. Amplification of the signal involves both phosphatidylinositol (PI) and inositol triphosphate (IP$_3$), and induces a molecular cascade that results in smooth muscle relaxation and a number of longer-term metabolic responses, including the induction of both smooth muscle hypertrophy and hyperplasia

mechanism. Signal transduction results in G-protein-linked activation of phospholipase C (PL-C) and the donation of a high-energy phosphate molecule from GTP. Signal amplification is accomplished by a molecular cascade, involving phosphatidylinositol (PI) and inositol triphosphate (IP$_3$), which results in an influx of intracellular calcium producing smooth muscle contractions as well as activation of protein kinase C which, in turn, induces other intracellular metabolic responses[10] (Figure 17).

Causes of abnormal prostate cell growth

Two of the three dominant pathologies affecting the prostate gland, namely, BPH and prostate cancer, are characterized by abnormal cell proliferation. Prostatitis, however, is an inflammatory disorder. In BPH, the proliferative process affects both epithelial and stromal cells of the TZ. In contrast, prostate cancer is found more commonly in the PZ, where it arises from atypical luminal cells [prostatic intraepithelial neoplasia (PIN)].

Abnormal cell growth in both BPH and prostate cancer may, in part, be the result of activation of oncogenes. Several of these have been implicated in the pathogenesis of prostate cancer and it is not implausible that they may also underlie the benign proliferative process of BPH.

Oncogenes

The *ras* proto-oncogene is normally involved in the regulation of cell growth and division. A mutation (Figure 18A) resulting in a single base-pair change causes an inability to separate GTP from the *ras* p21 protein, thereby locking it permanently in its activated form. The result is a continuing signal for cell proliferation (Figure 18B).

Another oncogene, c-*erb* B-2, acts through a different mechanism. A point mutation of DNA segment coding for c-*erb* B-2 results in the production of a distorted version of the EGF receptor. This mutant protein has no external component, with the result that the internal component continually signals the need for cell division regardless of the presence or absence of EGF signal molecules[11] (Figure 19).

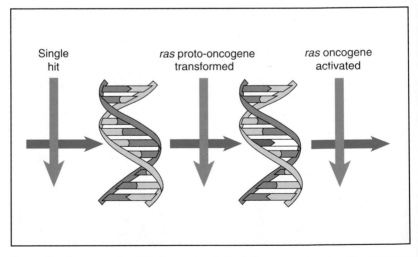

Figure 18A Oncogenesis within the prostate is due to the conversion of proto-oncogenes to active oncogenes. In the case of the *ras* oncogene, this occurs as a result of a mutation, or 'hit', involving alteration of a single nucleotide base pair

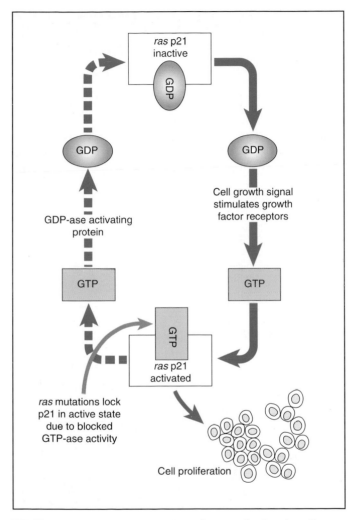

Figure 18B The mutated *ras* oncogene p21 protein cannot be deactivated by guanosine triphosphate (GTP) cyclase and thus continues to signal inappropriately for cell growth and division

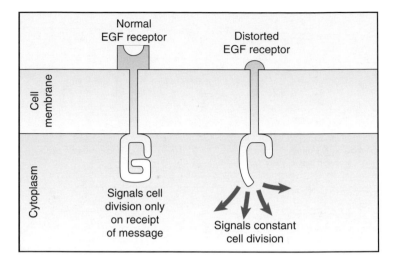

Figure 19 c-*erb* B-2 oncogene activation involves the production of truncated versions of the EGF receptor. The truncated receptor signals for continued cell growth and division regardless of the presence or absence of EGF signal molecules

Tumor suppressor genes

As well as the influence of growth-promoting oncogenes, abnormal prostate cell growth may also be the result of loss of the growth-restraining influences of one or more tumor suppressor genes[12], the best examples of which are the p53 and retinoblastoma tumor suppressor genes[13,14]. The p53 protein encoded by the former gene acts as an important regulator of cell division. Point mutation or complete deletion of this gene allows abnormal cell proliferation to occur (Figure 20).

Alterations of the p53 tumor suppressor gene have also been implicated as one of the important step-wise mutations which result in the development of other cancers, including lung, breast, colon and bladder neoplasms[15,16].

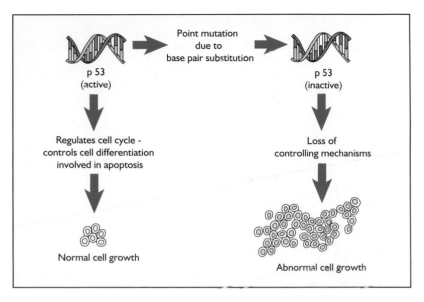

Figure 20 Tumor suppressor genes such as p53 are also important in the development of prostatic neoplasia. Normally, the p53 protein is involved in the regulation of cell division. Mutation or deletion of the gene thus encourages uncontrolled cell division

Pathology of the prostate

Accurate histological identification of the three basic pathological processes – adenocarcinoma, BPH and prostatitis – that affect the prostate is central to accurate diagnosis and correct institution of therapy. Whereas a detailed exposition of the many unusual variations of prostatic pathology are beyond the scope of this Pocketbook, the classical appearances of the most prevalent disorders are exemplified here.

Benign prostatic hyperplasia

Histological BPH is classically characterized by a mixed proliferation of both stromal and epithelial elements to form nodules (Figures 21 and 22). There are, however, individual variations, with some patients developing a predominantly stromal version of the disease and others showing mainly epithelial overgrowth (Figure 23).

The luminal-to-basal cell relationship is retained in epithelial hyperplasia, which is not considered to be a premalignant condition. Subgroups of epithelial hyperplasia include basal cell (Figure 24) and cribriform hyperplasia. However, their only importance is the occasional difficulty in distinguishing them from cancer.

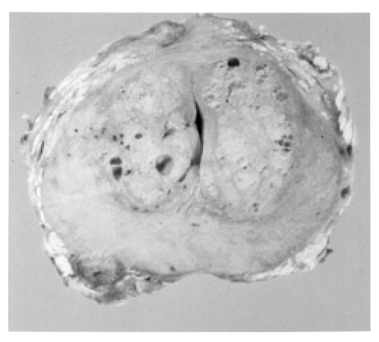

Figure 21 Transverse section of a prostate (5 cm across) showing bilateral hyperplastic nodules which have reduced the urethra to a slit. In contrast, the carcinoma is seen as solid homogeneous tissue posteriorly (on the right)

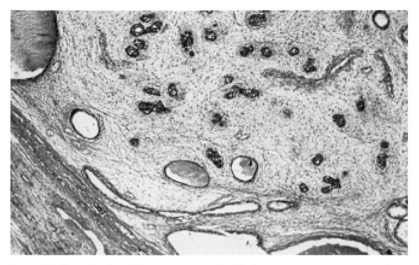

Figure 22 Hyperplastic nodules, composed of epithelium and stroma, can be seen here compressing the adjacent gland. (H & E)

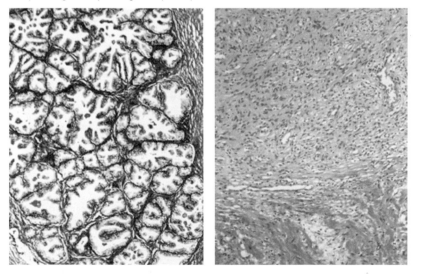

Figure 23 Hyperplastic nodules may be due to either predominantly epithelial (left) or stromal (right) overgrowth. Stromal nodules are almost always periurethral and are often situated immediately beneath the urethral epithelium. (H & E)

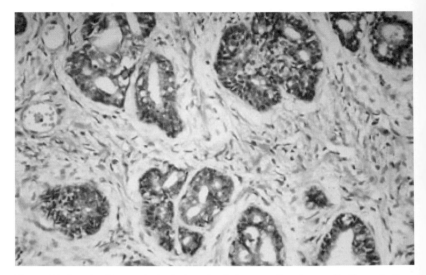

Figure 24 Basal cell hyperplasia: the basal cells have produced a stratified layer that has compressed the tall columnar cells into a narrow rim. These small hyperchromatic acini may be misdiagnosed as cancer, but the double-cell layer (comprising LP34-positive outer basal cells and compressed PSA-positive luminal cells) confirms the benign nature of this appearance. (H & E)

Prostate cancer

There is now convincing evidence to suggest that many prostate cancers are preceded by a preinvasive malignant change in the luminal cells known as prostatic intraepithelial neoplasia (PIN)[17]. The condition is characterized by progressive dysplasia of the prostatic epithelium initially within an intact basal cell layer. PIN was initially subdivided into mild, moderate and severe forms[18], but the terms 'low-grade' and 'high-grade' are now widely used[19] (Figures 25 and 26).

Essential for the diagnosis of prostatic carcinoma, as opposed to PIN, is the demonstration of invasion: carcinoma lacks basal cells whereas PIN may have an intact or intermittent basal cell layer, as the tendency of neoplastic prostatic epithelial cells is to invade the basement membrane. Identification of this process of invasion can be facilitated by the use of cytokeratin immunocytochemistry to delineate basal cells (Figure 27; see also Figure 6).

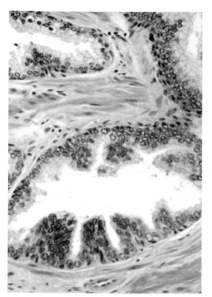
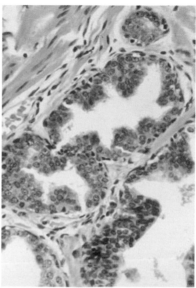

Figure 25 Low-grade prostatic intraepithelial neoplasia (PIN; lower field): The luminal epithelium is stratified and the nuclei are larger than that of the normal acinus (upper field). (H & E)

Figure 26 High-grade PIN: the luminal epithelium is stratified, but the cells have lost their polarity. The nuclei are larger than normal and contain nucleoli. In this section, an outer layer of basal cells can still be seen. (H & E)

Once invasion has occurred, the histological grading of the malignancy is best accomplished by use of the Gleason's technique[20] which is based on the tendency of a given tumor to form gland-like structures (Figure 28). Because of the marked heterogeneity of prostatic cancers, the Gleason score is calculated as the sum of the grades of the two dominant histological patterns within a given cancer.

Gleason grades 1–4 are well differentiated (Figures 29 and 30), grades 5–7 are moderately well differentiated (Figures 31 and 32) and grades 7–10 are poorly differentiated varieties of prostate cancer. These tumor gradings appear to correlate well with subsequent metastatic potential and overall survival. Cancers originating in the TZ tend to have a lower Gleason grade than tumors of the PZ, an observation which correlates well with the higher proliferative rates seen in the latter.

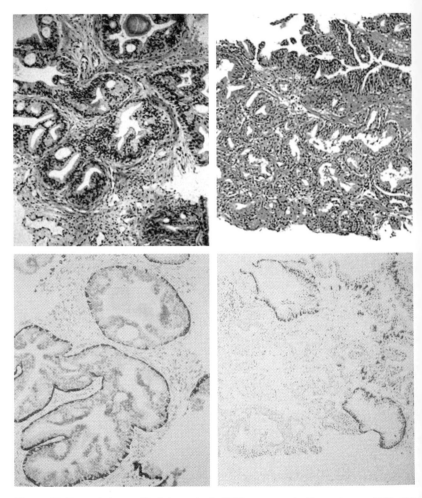

Figure 27 Prostatic intraepithelial neoplasia (PIN) compared with carcinoma: PIN may resemble cancer architecturally and/ or cytologically (upper left) with H & E staining, but can be shown to have a basal cell layer (lower left) immunocytochemically whereas, with carcinoma (upper right), the basal cell layer cannot be demonstrated (lower right); the positive staining is found only in residual benign ducts or acini

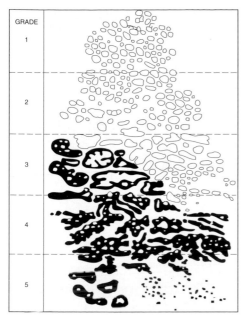

Figure 28 The Gleason grading system is the most widely used system for grading prostatic adenocarcinoma. Devised during the Veterans Administration Cooperative Urological Research Group studies (1960–75), different tumor patterns were identified without preconceived rating. Their presence was recorded and subsequently correlated with survival data by the study statistician. The patterns were arranged into five grades, numbered in order of increasing malignancy as determined by the mortality data.

The methodology has stood the test of time. As prostatic adenocarcinoma is morphologically heterogeneous and does not appear to be "as bad as its worst part", but behaves in accordance to its average morphology, the two dominant grades are identified and summated to arrive at a Gleason score (for example, grade 3 + grade 2 = Gleason score 5) for a given patient

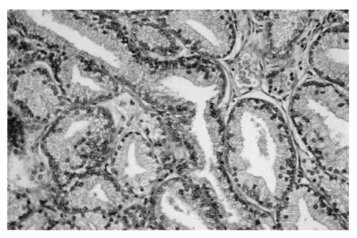

Figure 29 Gleason grade 2: this is characterized by small acini of varying diameter. Gleason grade 1 is similar, but has acini which are more consistent in size and form nodules with a well-defined edge

33

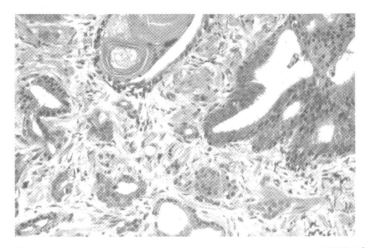

Figure 30 Gleason grade 3: these are typically small, angular, malignant acini that form an irregular mass and infiltrate benign acini at the edge of the lesion. In this section, there is a benign acinus containing corpora amylacea (top of field); PIN is also present (on the right)

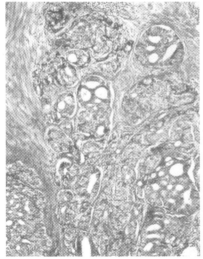

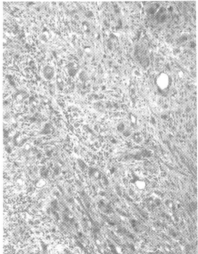

Figure 31 Gleason grade 4: the malignant acini fuse to form irregular masses, often with a cribriform result. A clear-celled 'hypernephroid' form is also described in this grading

Figure 32 Gleason grade 5: this is characterized by sheets of malignant cells with little evidence of gland formation. Single-celled infiltration is common

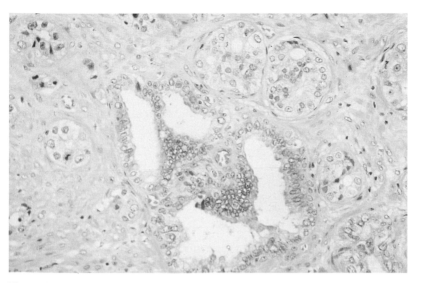

Figure 33 Adenocarcinoma can be seen spreading into a seminal vesicle. The benign epithelium of the vesicle can be seen centrally

Further information concerning the biological aggressiveness of the cancer can be gleaned from features such as perineural invasion, infiltration of adipose tissue or striated muscle and seminal vesicle invasion (Figure 33). A new technique which shows promise as a predictor of tumor stage is neo-vascularity[21], which gives an indication of the tumor's angiogenic activity.

Histology of prostate metastases

Most prostate cancer metastases are readily identifiable as being consistent with the previously diagnosed prostatic primary. However, in those patients in whom metastases are the presenting feature, or where the secondary deposit is poorly differentiated, then immunocytochemical detection of PSA is often invaluable (Figure 34).

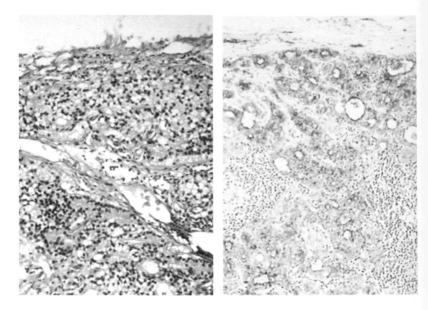

Figure 34 An adenocarcinoma can be seen infiltrating a lymph node from the obturator fossa with H & E staining (left) and with immunocytochemical preparation to demonstrate PSA (right)

Bladder outlet obstruction

Benign prostatic hyperplasia, prostate cancer and acute or chronic prostatitis may all result in bladder outlet obstruction (BOO). In addition, other non-prostatic disorders, such as bladder neck dyssynergia and urethral stricture disease (Figure 35), may also result in BOO. In response to the changes associated with increased outflow resistance, the detrusor muscle undergoes hypertrophy with the development of trabeculations and bladder wall thickening.

Although bladder wall hypertrophy, which develops in response to the increased effort required during voiding, is associated with an increase in size and strength of detrusor smooth muscle bundles, there is also infiltration by collagen (Figure 36) and a relative depletion of parasympathetic nerve endings. Thus, the overall efficiency of bladder contraction may be impaired, leading to the progressive development of post-void residual urine (PVR) and eventually acute chronic urinary retention.

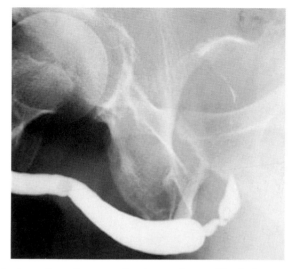

Figure 35 A retrograde urethrogram showing a stricture of the bulbar urethra. In older men, the bladder outflow obstruction resulting from such a stricture may mimic obstructive BPH

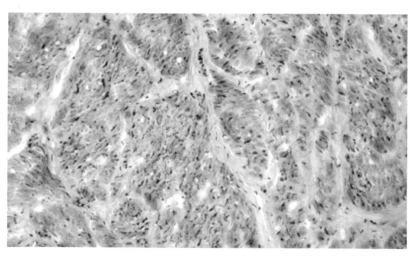

Figure 36 Collagen deposition has occurred between the smooth muscle cell bundles of the bladder detrusor muscle. This phenomenon is seen as part of the bladder response to the gradual development of obstruction. (Masson trichrome)

37

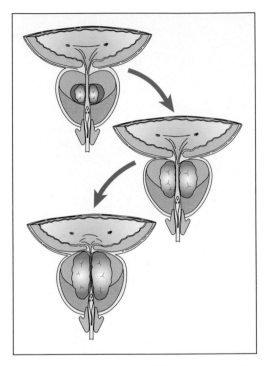

Figure 37 The progressive development of BPH tissue in the transition zone of the prostate results in gradually increasing bladder outflow obstruction

Progressive development of benign prostatic hyperplasia

As suggested by Berry *et al.*[22] on the basis of autopsy studies, BPH is generally a gradually progressive disease that commences in men who are around 40 years of age. Data from the Baltimore Longitudinal Study of Aging[23] suggest that symptomatic BPH also tends to progress with time in the majority of men. The average prostate volume increase is in the order of 0.6 ml/year, and this is associated with a mean diminution of flow rate of 0.2 ml/s/year[24].

The explanation for these findings lies in the progressive expansion of the TZ by the adenoma (Figure 37). This process reduces the distensibility of the urethra during voiding and produces gradually increasing BOO.

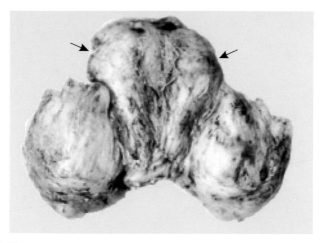

Figure 38 This specimen, removed at open operation, shows enlargement of both so-called lateral lobes as well as of the middle lobe (arrowed)

The anatomical distribution of the adenoma is not always uniform. When the process affects mainly the proximal periurethral zone, so-called median or middle lobe enlargement occurs (Figure 38). In this situation, the adenoma is often stromal rather than glandular in nature, is not detectable by digital rectal examination (DRE) and is commonly associated with a disproportionate amount of BOO. Recently, it has been observed that larger glands have faster growth rates than smaller prostates. This may help to explain why men with larger glands are at greater risk of acute urinary retention (AUR).

Localized progression of prostate cancer

Most prostate cancers probably start as PIN and develop into well-differentiated lesions in the PZ of the prostate. They grow slowly at first, often with a cell-doubling time of more than 2 years. As dedifferentiation occurs due to sequential mutations, however, the cell division rate increases and local invasion occurs.

The TNM (tumors/nodes/metastases) staging system classifies prostate cancers locally as T1–4 (Figure 39). Impalpable tumors, which are now being detected with increasing frequency, are classified as T1A and T1B

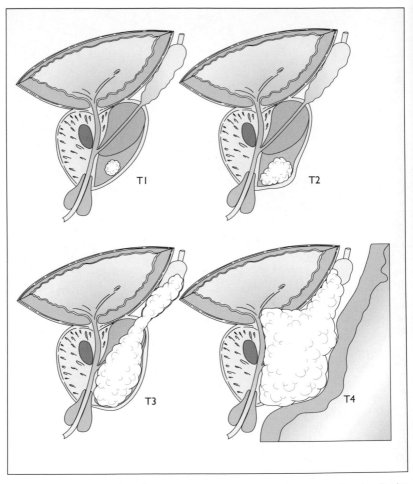

Figure 39 Clinical staging of prostate cancer: most prostate cancers develop in the peripheral zone and, when sufficiently large, become palpable as a T2 lesion. A T3 lesion denotes invasion of the prostatic capsule, and a T4 lesion often involves either the seminal vesicles or other adjacent structures

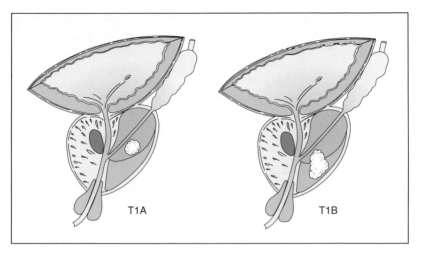

Figure 40 Impalpable prostate cancer is not infrequently diagnosed at the time of transurethral resection of the prostate (TURP). If the cancer is well differentiated and involves less than 5% of the resected material, it is classed as a T1A and carries a good prognosis. If, on the other hand, the lesion is moderately or poorly differentiated and involves more than 5% of the resected chippings, then it is termed a T1B lesion. These lesions are associated with a poorer prognosis and a higher probability that residual cancer will persist in the prostate remnant after resection and require further therapy

(according to grade and volume) when identified by transurethral resection (TUR; Figure 40), or as T1C if impalpable, and detected by an elevated PSA and subsequent transrectal ultrasound (TRUS)-guided biopsy.

Local extension of prostate adenocarcinoma most frequently occurs through the capsule (so-called capsular extension) posterolaterally via lymphatics, which follow the prostatic branches of the neurovascular bundles of Walsh (Figures 41 and 42). For this reason, it is generally advised that, during a nerve-sparing radical retropubic prostatectomy, the neurovascular bundle on the affected side be sacrificed to reduce the chances of a positive surgical margin in that location.

Further local extension most commonly involves the seminal vesicles, a pathological finding which is associated with a poor prognosis (see Figure 33). Prostatic tumor may also infiltrate the bladder base and obstruct the ureteric orifices, producing hydronephrosis and, if bilateral, eventual anuria.

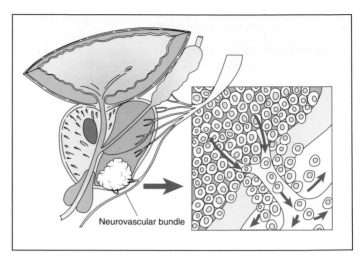

Neurovascular bundle

Figure 41 Because many prostate cancers develop posteriorly in the peripheral zone of the gland, it is not surprising that tumor cells are often able to escape the confines of the gland through the veins and lymphatics that accompany the neurovascular bundles of Walsh

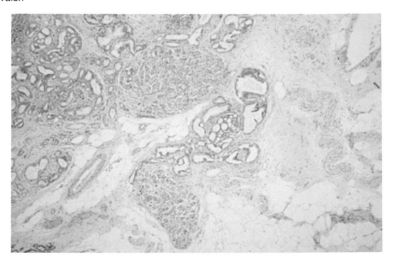

Figure 42 An adenocarcinoma can be seen extending posterolaterally beyond the gland into adipose tissue to encircle the neighboring nerves and ganglia. Perineural invasion must be considered during nerve-sparing surgery if positive margins are to be avoided

Metastatic spread of prostate cancer

The favored sites of prostate cancer metastases (Figure 43) are the obturator lymph nodes and the bony skeleton. However, lymph nodes elsewhere, the lungs and other soft tissues may also be involved.

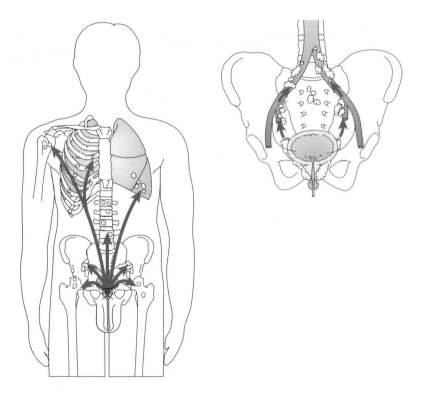

Figure 43 The favored sites of metastases from prostate cancer are the lymphatic nodes of the obturator fossa and the bony skeleton, in particular, the dorsolumbar spine and bony pelvis

Diagnosis of prostatic diseases

History

Because the prostate surrounds the urethra, patients who have prostatic diseases most frequently complain of micturition-related symptoms. These have been subdivided into irritative (storage) and obstructive (voiding) symptoms. Irritative symptoms have the most impact on the patient's QoL.

To quantitate the severity of symptoms, a numerical symptom-scoring system was first devised by a subcommittee of the American Urological Association (AUA)[25,26] and then adopted by the International Consensus Committee (ICC) as the International Prostate Symptom Score (IPSS). As an adjunct to the symptom score, there is also a single question that attempts to evaluate the impact of the symptoms on the QoL.

Other symptoms that are suggestive of prostatic or bladder disease, but which are not encompassed by the IPSS, include perineal pain, hematuria, dysuria, hemospermia and, in the case of metastatic prostate cancer, sudden onset of lower back or pelvic pain.

Physical examination

A general physical examination, including blood pressure measurement, is important in all patients with prostatic disease as men beyond middle age not uncommonly harbor other co-morbid conditions such as hypertension or chronic obstructive airways disease (COAD). A focused neurological examination will identify most significant neurological diseases which may be masquerading as prostatism. Palpation and percussion of the lower abdomen may reveal a chronically distended bladder due to chronic urinary retention.

The cornerstone of the physical examination in the patient with suspected prostatic disease is the digital rectal examination (DRE). This may be performed with the patient in the left lateral, knee-elbow or forward-bend position. A well-lubricated gloved finger is inserted into the rectum to evaluate the size and consistency of the gland.

The normal prostate should be the size of a chestnut and possess a springy consistency similar to that of the tip of the nose. The median sulcus is normally palpable, but the seminal vesicles should not be appreciable (Figure 44).

44

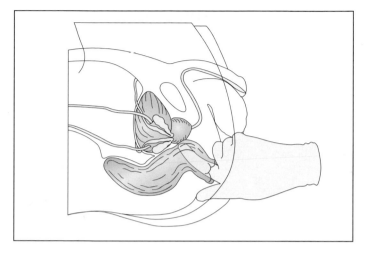

Figure 44 Digital rectal examination (DRE) allows the detection of posteriorly located tumors, which may be identified as an induration or distinct nodules, or as a cause of asymmetry of the gland

In prostatitis, the prostate may feel normal, boggy, tender or indurated on DRE. If a prostatic abscess is present, the gland becomes fluctuant and exquisitely tender. In BPH, the prostate is usually symmetrically enlarged and maintains its normal springy consistency. Bimanual examination in a relaxed patient may sometimes reveal either an unsuspected intravesical component of BPH or a chronically distended bladder.

DRE in patients suffering from prostate cancer may reveal a distinct nodule, diffuse induration or asymmetry of the gland. When the lesion involves the seminal vesicles, these structures may become palpable as firm 'cords' running superolaterally from the indurated prostate itself[27].

Microscopy and culture of urine, and expressed prostatic secretions

Urine microscopy and culture are important in most patients with lower urinary tract symptoms. Hematuria on microscopy may alert the clinician to coincidental pathology such as transitional cell carcinoma or carcinoma-in-situ. A positive urine culture with antibiotic sensitivities indicates the need for appropriate antibiotic therapy.

If prostatitis is suspected, culture and microscopy of expressed prostatic secretions (EPS) are indicated. The specimens must be carefully obtained (Figure 45) and bacteriological techniques capable of quantifying small

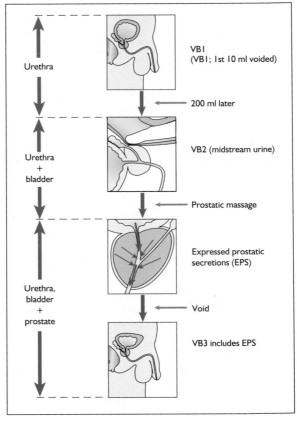

Figure 45 Bacterial prostatitis may be diagnosed by a lower tract localization (LTL) test. Initial and mid-stream urine specimens are collected and cultured; this is followed by a vigorous prostatic massage, after which an expressed prostatic secretion (EPS) sample is sent for culture. Finally, a further initial urine specimen is obtained and cultured. Differential bacterial counts among the various specimens may be an indication of an intra-prostatic infection

numbers of fastidious organisms, including facultative anaerobes such as *Ureaplasma urealyticum,* should be employed.

When the bladder urine is sterile, or nearly so, urethral colonization is indicated by a much higher count in the first-voided 10 ml of urine (voided bladder 1; VB1) than obtained from either EPS or the first-voided 10 ml of urine after prostatic massage (VB3). In contrast, with bacterial prostatitis, the bacterial count in the EPS and VB3 cultures should exceed those of the VB1 and VB2 cultures by at least a factor of 10 or more.

Serology

A blood urea nitrogen (BUN) and serum creatinine assay are usually requested in patients presenting with lower urinary tract symptoms. Around one in ten patients with BPH and/or prostate cancer have some elevation of serum creatinine, although this is not always the result of BOO *per se*. A full blood count occasionally reveals anemia or other clinically significant abnormalities such as leukocytosis.

The most important – and most controversial – serological test in prostatic disease is the PSA assay. Levels of this glycoprotein are elevated in diseases which interfere with the integrity of the basement membrane surrounding prostatic acini. In around one in ten patients with BPH, in the occasional patient with prostatitis or prostatic infarction (Figure 46) and in most patients with clinically significant volumes of prostate cancer, PSA values are greater than the upper limit of normal (4 ng/ml[28,29] with the most commonly employed Hybritech™ or Abbott IMX™ immunometric assays).

Recently, it has been discovered that differential assays comparing the ratio of free to complexed PSA may further help to discriminate between BPH and prostate cancer[30] (Figure 47). In patients with prostate cancer, a greater proportion of the serum PSA is bound to the protein antichymotrypsin (ACT) than in BPH, resulting in a reduction of the free-to-total PSA ratio.

Elevated total levels of PSA or reduction of the free-to-total PSA ratio may therefore act as a marker for as yet impalpable prostate cancer. In men whose life expectancy exceeds 10 years, earlier diagnosis of prostate cancer may allow curative treatment, and thus prevent local extension and/or the development of metastases. Theoretically at least, this should reduce

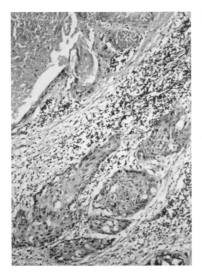

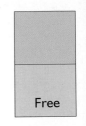

Advanced prostate cancer
Most of PSA
immunoreactivity has
a molecular size of
90 kDa

BPH
Most of PSA
immunoreactivity has
a molecular size of
30 kDa

Figure 46 This histological section shows an area of prostatic infarction (upper left) with characteristic squamous metaplasia of the adjacent acini. Prostatic infarction is associated with a rise in PSA and, occasionally, with the development of acute urinary retention. (H & E)

Figure 47 The ratio of free to total PSA is greater in BPH than in prostate cancer. With the use of a highly sensitive immunofluorometric assay, the concentration of serum free PSA in relation to PSA bound to the protein antichymotrypsin can be determined, which may help to differentiate between these two prostatic diseases

cancer-specific mortality, although this remains to be proved by long-term randomized studies of screening and early intervention which are ongoing.

Imaging studies and urinary flow rate determination

The combined use of imaging studies and uroflow measurement aims to identify both structural and functional abnormalities in the upper and lower urinary tract. The normal bladder fills from undilated kidneys and ureters to a volume of 300–500 ml and then empties completely through an unobstructed outlet at a maximum flow rate of more than 15 ml/s. A plain X-ray can identify radiopaque calculi in the bladder (Figure 48).

Contrast administered intravenously may demonstrate anatomical abnormalities in the upper tracts and, albeit with less sensitivity, in the bladder itself. Figure 49 is an intravenous urogram (IVU) showing the

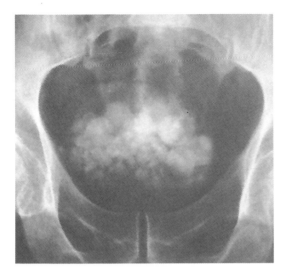

Figure 48 These multiple bladder stones, visualized on a plain abdominal X-ray, are sometimes seen in association with a benignly enlarged prostate

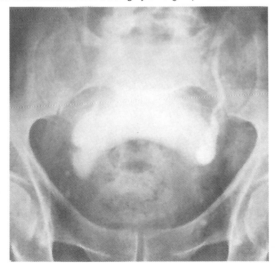

Figure 49 This intravenous urogram (IVU) shows a benign prostate gland which is sufficiently massive to cause an indentation of the base of the bladder. The adenoma weighed more than 200 g at the time of removal by retropubic prostatectomy

49

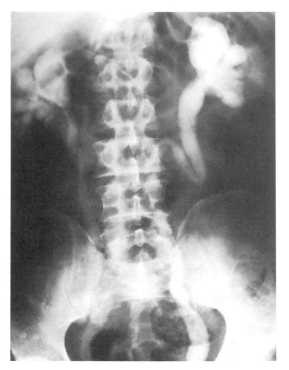

Figure 50 An IVU showing bilateral hydronephrosis secondary to BPH. The distal ends of the ureters are characteristically hook-shaped in appearance. If obstruction is relieved, this appearance will return to normal

typical IVU appearances of a large, benignly enlarged, prostate causing an indentation at the base of the bladder. In less than 2% of cases, the outflow obstruction due to BPH is severe enough to result in bilateral hydronephrosis (Figure 50). In contrast, in locally advanced prostate cancer, unilateral or bilateral ureteric obstruction is not uncommon and may be the result of either obstruction of the intramural ureter at the level of the trigone or constriction at the pelvic brim due to lymph node metastases (Figure 51).

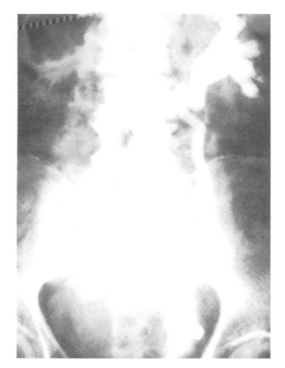

Figure 51 Nephrostogram showing left lower ureteric obstruction secondary to prostatic adenocarcinoma. The right kidney is non-functioning due to obstruction

Transabdominal ultrasound imaging

Transabdominal ultrasound imaging provides a simple, non-invasive and cost-effective means of imaging the bladder and prostate, and excludes upper tract dilatation. A pre- and post-void estimation of bladder volume allows evaluation of the PVR volume of urine, although several studies have shown that there is a marked void-to-void variation in the values recorded[31]. Median lobe enlargement of the prostate is readily visualized (Figure 52), but the architecture of the posterior portion and TZ of the gland are best imaged by an endocavity transrectal ultrasound probe.

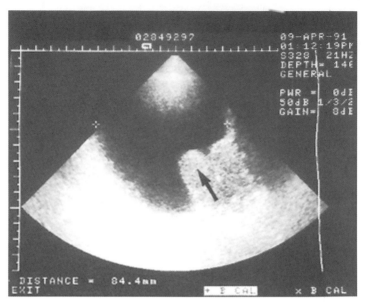

Figure 52 Transabdominal ultrasound showing pronounced indentation of the bladder due to considerable BPH with median lobe enlargement (arrowed)

Uroflowmetry

Most, if not all, patients with prostatic disease require uroflowmetry to quantitate objectively the severity of their BOO. A voided volume of more than 150 ml is required to achieve a reliable recording. With this proviso, the test has an acceptable test–retest reproducibility[32]. Patients should be advised to avoid abdominal straining during the measurement, as this may result in artefactual peaks, and should feel that the bladder is full prior to the test. Figures 53 and 54 are examples of a normal and an obstructed uroflow trace, respectively.

Maximum uroflow values are the most clinically useful single parameter. Values above 15 ml/s have an approximately 70% probability of obstruction, whereas values below 10 ml/s are associated with a urodynamic BOO in more than 90% of cases.

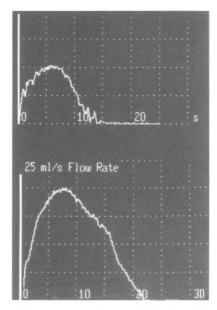

Figure 53 These two uroflowmetry recordings were both taken in the same unobstructed patient, one at a volume of 100 ml, the other with a voided volume of 350 ml. The apparent discrepancy demonstrates the dependence of uroflow measurements on adequate prevoiding bladder filling

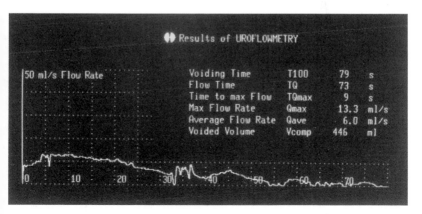

Figure 54 This uroflow recording from a patient with bladder outflow obstruction secondary to BPH shows a reduced maximum flow and prolonged voiding

Transrectal ultrasound imaging

Transrectal ultrasound (TRUS) imaging of the prostate serves several purposes:

- Imaging the internal architecture of the gland;
- Determination of prostate volume;
- Facilitation of ultrasound-guided prostate biopsy.

A 7-MHz endocavity ultrasound probe is usually used and the prostate viewed in both anteroposterior (AP) and sagittal planes (Figures 55 and 56). BPH is characterized by hypoechoic expansion of the TZ[33] (Figure 57). Adenocarcinomata are sometimes visualized as hypoechoic foci (and less often as hyperechoic) most usually in the PZ (Figures 58 and 59) and less frequently at the apex of the gland[34] (Figure 60). Many smaller prostate

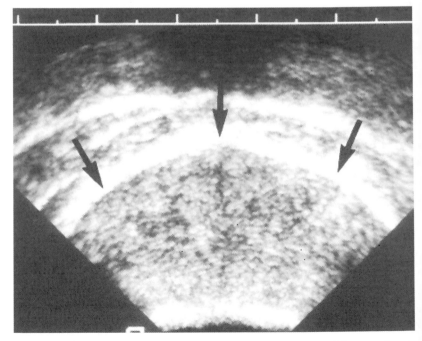

Figure 55 Transrectal ultrasound (TRUS) showing the appearances of the normal prostate in anteroposterior view

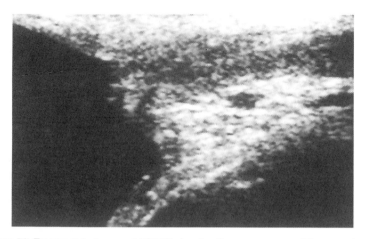

Figure 56 Transrectal ultrasound (TRUS) showing the appearances of the normal prostate in sagittal view

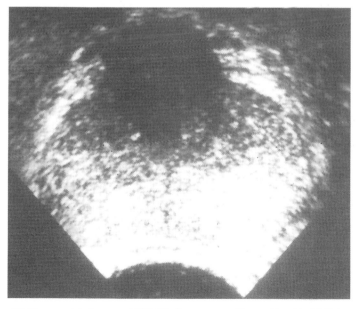

Figure 57 Transrectal ultrasound (TRUS) of a prostate with considerable BPH showing a characteristically large periurethral hypoechoic area (anteroposterior view)

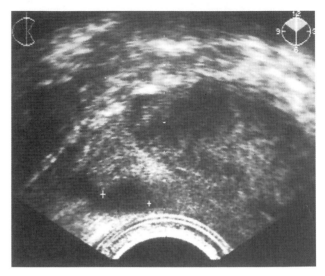

Figure 58 Transrectal ultrasound (TRUS) showing a hypoechoic area in the peripheral zone which proved, on biopsy, to be an adenocarcinoma (anteroposterior view)

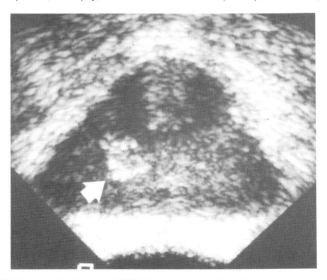

Figure 59 Transrectal ultrasound (TRUS) showing an atypical hyperechoic appearance (arrowed) of prostate cancer

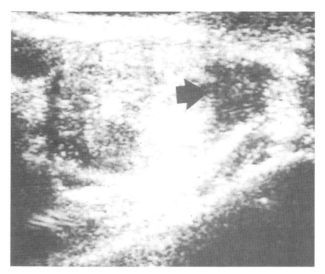

Figure 60 Transrectal ultrasound (TRUS) showing a hypoechoic adenocarcinoma at the apex of the gland (arrowed)

cancers, however, are isoechoic and can be identified only by systematic sextant biopsy.

On occasions, TRUS allows estimation of the local stage of a prostate cancer because asymmetry and irregularity of the capsule are associated with extracapsular spread of adenocarcinoma[35].

The advent of color Doppler ultrasound imaging (CDI) and its incorporation into TRUS technology have allowed evaluation of prostatic blood flow. The main clinical value of this technology is in the imaging of patients with prostatitis, when objective confirmation of the inflammatory process may be helpful (Figure 61). Prostatic calculi, which may in themselves be the cause of prostatic inflammation, can sometimes be visualized (Figure 62) as a cause of obstruction to the ejaculatory ducts.

After administration of a covering dose of an antibiotic treatment, which should be continued for several days, systematic TRUS-guided biopsy of the prostate may be obtained (Figure 63). Biopsies are best after infiltration of the gland with local anesthetic; this markedly reduces the discomfort associated with the procedure.

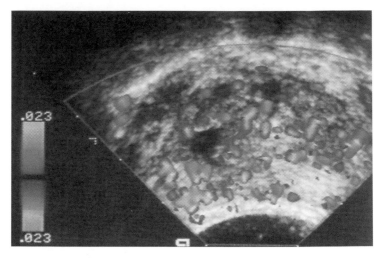

Figure 61 Color Doppler ultrasound of the prostate demonstrating increased vascularity due to acute prostatitis

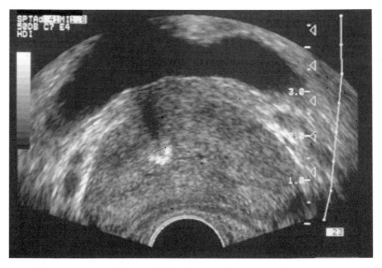

Figure 62 Transrectal ultrasound (TRUS) showing a prostatic calculus (arrowed) as a white patch. The calculus blocks the transmission of ultrasound waves, resulting in characteristic acoustic shadowing

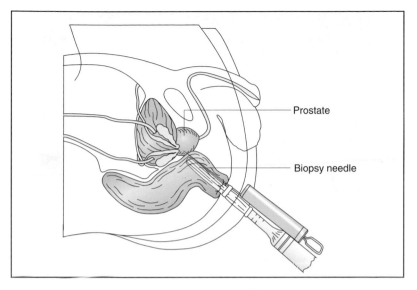

Figure 63 The procedure for TRUS-guided biopsy of the prostate should always be carried out under antibiotic cover, which should be continued for 3–4 days post-biopsy to reduce the incidence of infective complications. At present, the most common indications for biopsy are either an elevated PSA or a prostate that feels abnormal on DRE

Computed tomography and magnetic resonance imaging

Computed tomography (CT) and magnetic resonance imaging (MRI) are sometimes employed in the staging of prostatic cancer. Less frequently, these technologies are used to establish the precise volume of BPH present[36]. This can be helpful since men with larger glands are at greater risk of BPH progression.

CT scanning reveals the dimensions of the prostate, but does not clearly demonstrate its internal architecture (Figure 64). Irregularity of the gland may suggest the presence of extracapsular extension of tumor, but the sensitivity and specificity of this observation are low. CT scans are also employed to identify pelvic lymphadenopathy, usually an indication of metastatic spread but, even in such a situation, the accuracy is still low. In equivocal cases, CT guidance may allow fine-needle aspiration of enlarged lymph nodes for confirmatory cytological study (Figure 65).

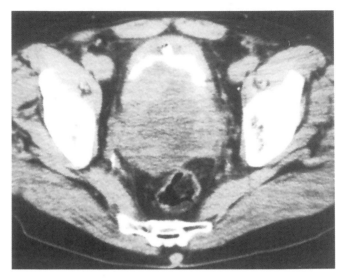

Figure 64 Although computed tomography (CT) scanning is able to demonstrate the prostate, visualization of the internal architecture is poor. Also, the use of this imaging modality for local staging is limited

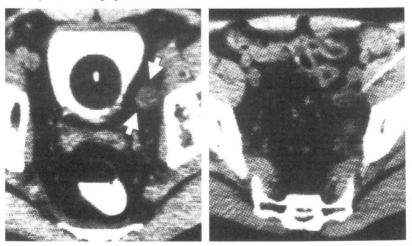

Figure 65 CT scanning can reveal pelvic lymphadenopathy (left), albeit with limited specificity, and can also be used to guide fine-needle aspiration (right) for cytological examination

Whole-body coils allow MRI imaging of the prostate, with which the PZ may be distinguished from the TZ (Figure 66). Adenocarcinoma may also be visualized by this means, although not all prostate cancers are as clearly demarcated from normal tissue as the example shown in Figure 67.

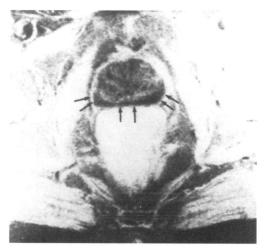

Figure 66 Magnetic resonance imaging (MRI) scan, using an external body coil, allows differentiation of the peripheral zone (arrowed) from the hyperplastic transitional zone

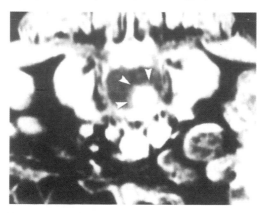

Figure 67 Magnetic resonance imaging (MRI) scan, using an external body coil, shows a peripherally located prostatic adenocarcinoma (arrowed)

Endorectal MRI provides more architectural detail of internal prostatic anatomy[37]. Figures 68 and 69 show T_1- and T_2-weighted images, respectively,

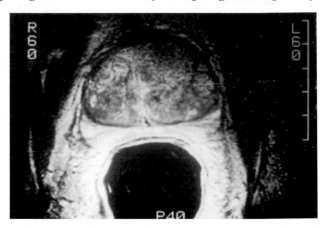

Figure 68 A T_1-weighted MRI scan, using an endorectal imaging coil, reveals an enlarged prostate showing changes of BPH

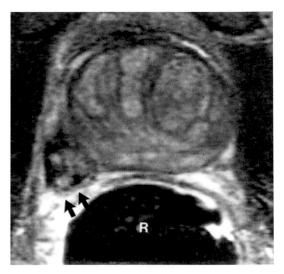

Figure 69 A T_2-weighted MRI scan, using an endorectal imaging coil, reveals a peripherally located prostatic adenocarcinoma (arrowed)

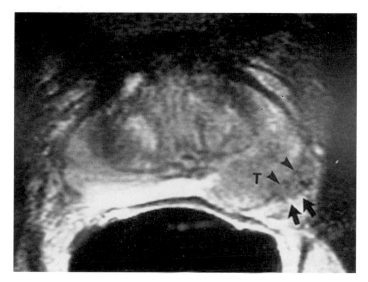

Figure 70 An endorectal MRI scan showing a peripherally located adenocarcinoma (arrowed) involving the neurovascular bundle on that side

of a prostate expanded by BPH tissue. Figure 70 is an MRI scan, taken with an endorectal coil, of a lesion in the PZ of the prostate that lies close to, and probably involves, the neurovascular bundle on the affected side.

MRI may also be useful in demonstrating lymph node metastases (Figure 71), or metastatic involvement of the spine (Figure 72), pelvis or long bones.

As MRI technology is advancing rapidly, we may anticipate even more precise and informative images in the future. The use of enhancing agents such as gadolinium has already produced improved results, and MRI spectroscopy seems likely to be the way ahead.

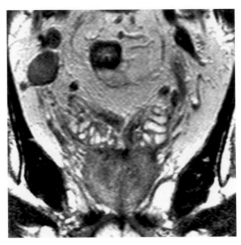

Figure 71 MRI scan showing lymph node enlargement (on the right) due to metastatic prostate cancer

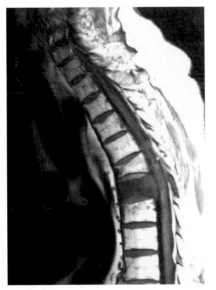

Figure 72 MRI scan of the thoracic spine showing involvement of one of the dorsal vertebral bodies by metastatic prostatic cancer. The adjacent vertebral body shows signs of collapse

Radionuclide bone scanning

Technetium radionuclide bone scanning has transformed our ability to detect early bone metastases from prostate cancer[38]. This technology, which is able to demonstrate clearly the abnormal vascularity in skeletal metastases, has a far higher sensitivity and specificity than the radiological skeletal surveys that it has now replaced.

Although bone scans are seldom positive in patients with PSA values below 20 ng/ml[39], they may be useful as a baseline in newly diagnosed cases because they allow documentation of false-positive areas due to other disease processes, such as osteoarthrosis of the spine or Paget's disease.

The most common appearance of prostate cancer metastases on a bone scan is as multiple 'hot spots', mainly affecting the lumbosacral spine and pelvis (Figures 73 and 74). The long bones and skull, however, may also be involved.

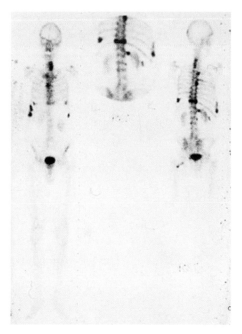

Figure 73 A radionuclide bone scan showing multiple metastatic deposits due to adeno-carcinoma of the prostate

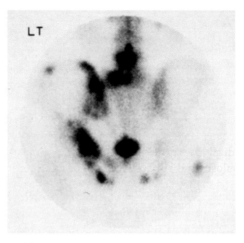

Figure 74 A radionuclide bone scan showing 'hot spots' in the pelvis, an indication of metastatic prostate cancer

In very extensive metastatic disease, the bone scan may occasionally be misleading because of diffusely increased skeletal uptake, an appearance known as a 'superscan' (Figure 75).

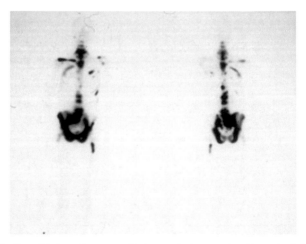

Figure 75 Radionuclide bone 'superscan' is the result of very extensive metastatic prostate cancer

Treatment options

Benign prostatic hyperplasia

BPH therapy has evolved over the last two decades from a simple choice between watchful waiting and transurethral resection of the prostate (TURP) to more complex decisions between available medical therapies and a considerable range of minimally invasive treatment options. Most patients with a degree of bother from their BPH-associated symptoms will now opt for medical therapy in the first instance. Alpha-blockers, such as doxazosin, tamsulosin and alfuzosin, can all be administered once per day and produce rapid and sustainable improvement of lower urinary tract symptoms and uroflow (Figure 76)[40]. The 5α-reductase inhibitor finasteride at a dose of 5 mg per day reduces prostate volume by around 20% and improves symptoms and uroflow almost as much as the α-blockers, but only after a 3–6-month initial treatment period[41]. Available evidence

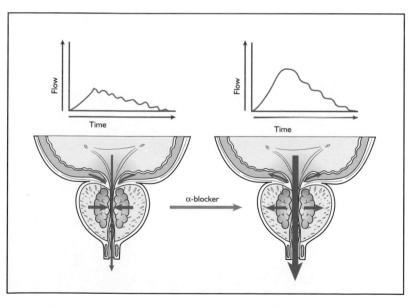

Figure 76 Mechanism of action of α-blockers: relaxation of the gland enhances flow rate and improves BPH-related symptoms

suggests that finasteride works most effectively in men with a clinically enlarged prostate and a PSA value >1.4 ng/ml[42]. The Proscar Long-term Efficacy and Safety Study (PLESS) has demonstrated that finasteride can reduce BPH-associated complications such as acute urinary retention (AUR) and the need for prostate surgery by more than 50%[43]. This beneficial impact of medical therapy on BPH progression has been confirmed by the Medical Therapy of Prostate Symptoms (MTOPS) study[44], which has been recently reported. In this 4.5-year trial, the combination of finasteride and doxazosin was significantly more effective than either agent alone or identical placebo in terms of preventing BPH progression.

Surgical treatment options are now mainly employed in men who have failed to respond to medical therapy or in those with complications of BPH such as AUR. TURP under either an epidural or a light general anesthetic still constitutes the gold standard (Figure 77); however, newer technologies such as Holmium laser resection, interstitial laser therapy and microwave thermotherapy are all producing increasingly promising results. Most surgical approaches have a negative impact on ejaculation, but leave erections and sensation of orgasm unaffected. This effect is not usually too troublesome provided that the patient has been counseled in advance.

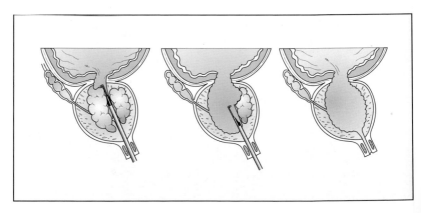

Figure 77 Transurethral resection of the prostate (TURP): a resectoscope is used to remove the obstructing transition zone tissue

Prostate cancer

Early disease: The management of early prostate cancer is one of the most controversial areas of prostate disease, and is likely to remain so until the results of the randomized controlled trials currently underway are available[45]. These trials include the Scandinavian trial comparing radical prostatectomy to external beam radiotherapy (EBRT) and the PIVOT trial comparing radical prostatectomy to watchful waiting. A new trial comparing radical prostatectomy with brachytherapy is planned.

Patients with clinically localized prostate cancer (i.e. biopsy-proven disease with no evidence of extra-prostatic extension) should be informed about the pros and cons of the following treatment options:

1. **Watchful waiting**: This option is most applicable in men with low-volume, less aggressive disease and in those with a life expectancy of less than 10 years. Regular PSA determinations are recommended and active treatment if disease progression occurs.
2. **Radical prostatectomy**: Considered by many to constitute the gold standard treatment, radical prostatectomy involves the removal of the entire prostate either retropubically, perineally or laparoscopically (Figure 78). Provided that all cancer tissue is excised (i.e. all surgical

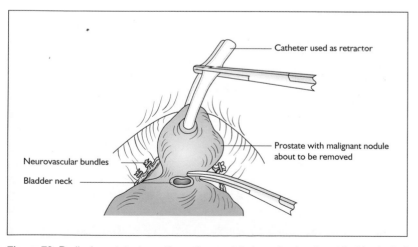

Catheter used as retractor

Prostate with malignant nodule about to be removed

Neurovascular bundles

Bladder neck

Figure 78 Radical prostatectomy: the entire prostate is excised and sent for histological examination

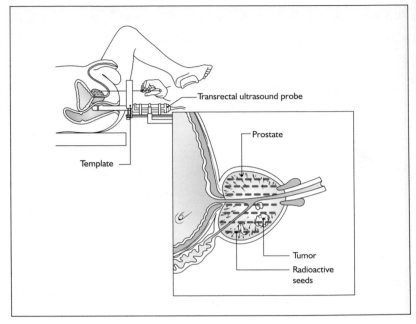

Figure 79 Brachytherapy: radioactive seeds are inserted transperineally into the prostate

margins and lymph nodes are clear), then life expectancy is equivalent
to that of an age-matched individual who has never suffered cancer.
Side-effects include a low risk (2–3%) of stress incontinence but a
higher (>50%) risk of erectile dysfunction, even when nerve-sparing
techniques are employed. However, both these problems can now be
treated effectively.

3. **External beam radiotherapy**: EBRT can provide an effective form of
    therapy for early prostate cancer. Results have been shown to be
    enhanced by the use of neo-adjuvant androgen ablation, usually with a
    luteinizing hormone releasing hormone (LHRH) analog. Side-effects
    include proctitis and rectal bleeding due to inclusion of the anterior
    rectal wall in the treatment field.

4. **Brachytherapy**: Brachytherapy involves the transperineal implanta-
    tion of radioactive seeds into the prostate under light anesthesia
    (Figure 79). Swelling of the gland in response may cause a worsening of

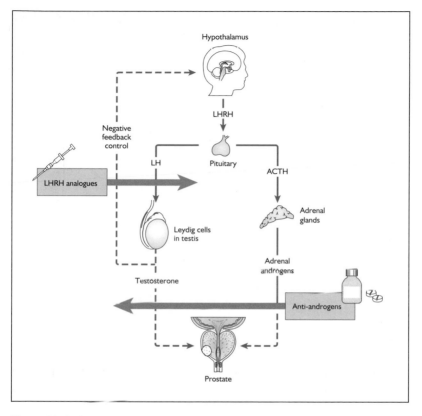

Figure 80 Androgen ablation therapy for prostate cancer: antiandrogens block both testicular and adrenal androgen stimulation of prostate tissues

lower urinary tract symptoms for some time. As a consequence, this form of treatment should be used with caution in patients with pre-existing bladder outflow obstruction.

Advanced disease: Patients with prostate cancer involving either regional lymph nodes or the bony skeleton are described as suffering from advanced disease. In either circumstance, cure is not possible; however androgen withdrawal will, in most cases, result in a remission that is maintained for on average 24–36 months, depending on the extent of the metastatic burden at presentation. Androgen ablation can be achieved either by bilateral orchidectomy or the use of depot LHRH analogs (Figure 80). Antiandrogens such as bicalutamide spare some aspects of sexual function, but are not as effective as the previously mentioned forms of androgen withdrawal when metastases are present.

Hormone-independent prostate cancer: Eventually, as a result of the selection of androgen-independent clones of cancer cells, prostate cancer sufferers treated by androgen ablation undergo disease relapse. In this situation, the first step is to withdraw any antiandrogen as this may result in a transient improvement of PSA values. Second-line treatments include either the use of oral estrogens in combination with aspirin or intravenous chemotherapy. Remissions are unfortunately short-lived but several newer approaches, such as the use of tyrosine kinase inhibitors and angiogenesis inhibitors, are currently under investigation.

Prostatitis

The treatment of prostatitis remains somewhat unsatisfactory. In the presence of documented prostatic infection, treatment with antibiotics is logical, and these may need to be continued for 6 weeks or longer. Even if expressed prostatic secretions are negative, response to antibiotics may be seen, especially if these are used in combination with anti-inflammatory agents. When a prostatic abscess is present, this may need to be drained transurethrally, and the pus cultured to determine appropriate antibiotic sensitivities. Chronic prostatitis has a very marked tendency to relapse, and patients should be warned of this and informed that further courses of treatment may become necessary.

Concluding perspectives

Quite suddenly, prostatic diseases seem to have come of age. The level of public interest has risen swiftly and with it the opportunities for research funding. This, in tandem with the recent explosive development of molecular biology, has produced new insights into the causes of BPH, prostate cancer and prostatitis. For example, a hereditary factor in the pathogenesis of prostate cancer has been localized to a region of the long arm of chromosome 1[46].

New consensus has now been reached concerning the diagnosis of prostatic diseases. PSA testing, although still controversial as a screening tool, is now established as a means of early detection as well as staging. Ultrasound studies, guided biopsy and bone scans provide the cornerstone of the diagnosis of prostatic cancer. Neither BPH nor prostatitis require biopsy confirmation. Ultrasound studies and flow rate measurement suffice for the former, while culture of expressed prostatic secretions is required for prostatitis.

BPH therapy has seen a shift from surgery to medical therapy. Alpha-blockers[40] and 5α-reductase inhibitors both appear safe and effective. The latter also have an important preventative effect against disease progression[43].

While treatment of advanced prostate cancer is generally agreed upon, therapy for localized prostate malignancy is much more controversial[45]. In the absence of firm evidence from randomized controlled trials, the best we can do at present is explain carefully to patients the advantages and disadvantages of radical retropubic prostatectomy, radical radiotherapy, brachytherapy or watchful waiting[47].

Although great strides have been made in all these disease areas, much work remains to be done to improve the quality of life of BPH and prostatitis sufferers, and to reduce the death toll from prostate cancer. It is to be anticipated and hoped that the innovative work currently being undertaken in laboratories and clinics around the world will translate into improvement of the quality of life of the many millions of prostate sufferers around the world.

References

1. Lowsley OS. The development of the human prostate gland with reference to the development of other structures of the neck of the urinary bladder. *Am J Anat* 1912;13:299
2. McNeal J. Regional morphology and pathology of the prostate. *Am J Clin Pathol* 1968;49:347–57
3. McNeal JE. The zonal anatomy of the prostate. *Prostate* 1891;2:35–49
4. Wang M, Valenzuela L, Murphy G, Chu T. Purification of human prostate specific antigen. *Invest Urol* 1979;17:159–63
5. Oesterling J. Prostate specific antigen: A critical assessment of the most useful tumor marker for adenocarcinoma of the prostate. *J Urol* 1991;145: 907–23

6. Oesterling JJ, Jacobsen SJ, Chute CG, *et al*. Serum prostate-specific antigen in a community-based population of healthy men. *JAMA* 1993;270:860–4

7. Bartsch G, Muller H, Boerholzer M, Rohr H. Light microscopic stereological analysis of the normal human prostate and benign prostatic hyperplasia. *J Urol* 1979;122:487–91

8. Shapiro E, Hartanto V, Lepor H. Anti-desmin vs. anti-actin for quantifying the area density of prostatic smooth muscle. *Prostate* 1992;20:259–63

9. Lepor H, Gregerman M, Crosby M, Mostofi FK, Walsh PC. Precise localization of the autonomic nerves from the pelvic plexus to the corpora cavernosa: A detailed anatomical study of the adult male pelvis. *J Urol* 1985;133:207–12

10. Ruffolo R, Nichols A, Stadel J, Hieble J. Structure and function of alpha adrenoceptors. *Pharm Rev* 1991;43:475–505

11. Zhau HE, Wan DS, Zhou J, Miller GJ, von Eschenbach AC. Expression of c-*erb* B-2/*neu* proto-oncogene in human prostatic cancer tissues and cell lines. *Mol Carc* 1992;5:320–7

12. Linehan WM. Molecular genetics of tumor suppressor genes in prostate carcinoma: The challenge and the promise ahead. [Editorial]. *J Urol* 1992;147:808–9

13. Effert PJ, Neubauer A, Walther PJ, Liu ET. Alterations of the p53 gene are associated with the progression of a human prostate carcinoma. *J Urol* 1992;147:789–93

14. Bookstein R, Rio P, Madreperla SA, Hong FE. Promoter deletion and loss of retinoblastoma gene expression in human prostate carcinoma. *Proc Natl Acad Sci* 1990;87:7762–6

15. Hollstein M, Sidransky D, Vogelstein B, Harris B. p53 mutations in human cancers. *Science* 1991;253:49–53

16. Sarkar F, Sakr W, Li Y, Maloska JE. Analysis of retinoblastoma (RB) gene deletion in human prostatic carcinoma. *Prostate* 1992;21:145–52

17. Bostwick D, Pacelli A, Lopez-Beltran A. Molecular biology of prostatic intraepithelial neoplasia. *Prostate* 1996;29:117–34

18. Bostwick DG. Premalignant lesions of the prostate. *Semin Diag Pathol* 1988;5:240–53

19. Bostwick DG, Brawer MK. Prostatic intraepithelial neoplasia and early invasion in prostate cancer. *Cancer* 1987;59:778–94

20. Gleason DE Histologic grading and clinical staging of prostatic carcinoma. In: Tannenbaum M, ed. *Urologic Pathology: The Prostate*. Philadelphia: Lea & Febiger, 1977:171–98

21. Brawer MK, Deering RE, Brown M, Preston SD, Bigier SA. Predictors of pathologic stage in prostatic carcinoma. The role of neovascularity. *Cancer* 1994;73:678–87

22. Berry SJ, Coffey DS, Walsh PC, Ewing LL. The development of human benign prostatic hyperplasia with age. *J Urol* 1984;132:474–9

23. Arrighi H, Guess H, Metter E, Fozard J. Symptoms and signs of prostatism as risk factors for prostatectomy. *Prostate* 1990;16:253–61

24. Drach GW, Layton TN, Binard WJ. Male peak urinary flow rate: Relationship of volume voided and age. *J Urol* 1979;122:210–14

25. Barry M, Fowler F, O'Leary M, *et al*. The American Urological Association symptom index for benign prostatic hyperplasia. *J Urol* 1992;148:1549–57

26. Barry M, Fowler F, O'Leary M, Bruskewitz R, Holtgrewe H, Mebust W. Correlation of the American Urological Association symptom index with self–administered versions of the Madsen-Iversen, Boyarsky, and Maine Medical Assessment Program symptom indexes. *J Urol* 1992;148:1558–63

27. Chodak GW, Keller P, Schoenberg HW. Assessment of screening for prostate cancer using the digital rectal examination. *J Urol* 1989; 141:1136–8

28. Catalona W, Smith D, Ratliff T, *et al*. Measurement of prostate specific antigen in serum as a screening test for prostate cancer. *N Engl J Med* 1991;324:1156–61

29. Catalona W, Richie J, Ahmann F, *et al*. A multicenter examination of PSA and digital rectal examination for early detection of prostate cancer in 6,374 volunteers. *J Urol* 1993;149:412A

30. Lilja H, Christensson A, Dahlen U, *et al*. Prostate specific antigen in serum occurs predominantly in complex with alpha$_1$ antichemotrypsin. *Clin Chem* 1991;37:1618–25

31. Dunsmuir W, Feneley M, Corry D, Bryan J, Kirby R. The day-to-day variation (test–retest reliability) of residual urine measurement. *Br J Urol* 1996; 77:192–3

32. Feneley M, Dunsmuir W, Pearce J, Kirby R. Reproducibility of uroflow measurement: Experience during a double-blind, placebo-controlled study of doxazosin in benign prostatic hyperplasia. *Urology* 1996;47:658–63

33. Rickards D. Transrectal ultrasound. *Br J Urol* 1992;69:449–55

34. Rifkin M, Choi H. Implications of small, peripheral hypoechoic lesions in endorectal US of the prostate. *Radiology* 1988;166:619–22

35. Ohori M, Egawa S, Shinohara K, Wheeler T, Scardino P Detection of microscopic extracapsular extension prior to radical prostatectomy for clinically localised prostate cancer. *Br J Urol* 1994;74:72–9

36. Hricak H, Dooms C, Jeffery R, *et al*. Prostatic carcinoma assessment by clinical assessment, CT and MRI imaging. *Radiology* 1987;162:331–6

37. Cheisky MJ, Schnall MD, Seidmon EJ, Pollack HM. Use of endorectal surface coil magnetic resonance imaging for local staging of prostate cancer. *J Urol* 1993;150:391–5

38. Jorgensen T, Muller C, Kaalhus O, Danielsen H, Tveter K. Extent of disease based on bone scan: Important prognostic indicator for patients with metastatic prostate cancer. *Eur Urol* 1995;28:40–6

39. Chybowski FM, Larson-Keller JJ, Bergstralh EJ, *et al*. Predicting radionuclide bone scan findings in patients with newly diagnosed, un-

treated prostate cancer. Prostate-specific antigen is superior to all other clinical parameters. *J Urol* 1991;145:313

40. Kirby RS, Pool JL. Alpha adrenoceptor blockade in the treatment of benign prostatic hyperplasia: past present and future *Br J Urol* 1997;80:521–2

41. Ekman P. Maximal efficacy of finasteride is obtained within 6 months and maintained over 6 years. *Eur Urol* 1998;33:312–17

42. Roehrhorn CG, Boyle P, Bergner D, *et al*. Serum prostate-specific antigen and prostate volume predict long-term changes in symptoms and flow rate: results of a four-year randomized trial comparing finasteride versus placebo. *Urology* 1999;54:662–9

43. McConnell JD, Bruskevitz R, Walsh PC, *et al*. The effect of finasteride on the risk of acute urinary retention and the need for surgical treatment among men with benign prostatic hyperplasia. *N Engl J Med* 1998;338:557–63

44. McConnell JD. The long term effects of medical therapy on the progression of BPH: results of the MTOPS trial. *J Urol* 2002;167:265A

45. Kirby RS. Treatment options for early prostate cancer. *Urology* 1998;52:948–62

46. Smith JR, Freije D, Carpten JD, *et al*. Major susceptibility locus for prostate cancer on chromosome 1 suggested by genome-wide search. *Science* 1996;274:1371–5

47. Middleton RG, Thompson JM, Austerfield MS, *et al*. Prostate cancer clinical guidelines summary report on the management of clinically localised prostate cancer. *J Urol* 1995;154:2144–8

Index